Still.

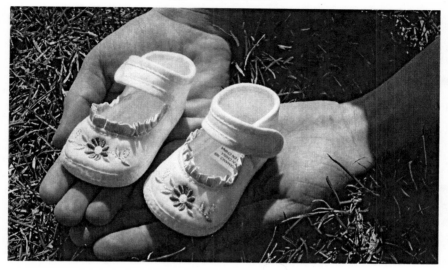

a collection of honest artwork and
writings from the heart of
a grieving mother

Stephanie Paige Cole

Eloquent Books

Eloquent Books
An imprint of Strategic Book Group
P.O. Box 333
Durham, CT 06422
www.StrategicBookGroup.com

ISBN: 978-1-60911-586-9

Dedication

This book, and all the work done by the Sweet Pea Project, is dedicated to the little girl who made me a mommy, my beautiful daughter Madeline Jonna Cole. Madeline gave me a lifetime of joy in an instant, and I will carry her with me in my heart forever. I am so grateful for the time we spent together and for all that she has given me. My life is richer and the world is a more beautiful place, because for forty-one weeks she was a part of it. Mommy loves you, Sweet Pea.

I would also like to thank my family for all their love and support. My husband Richy, for helping me keep my head above water even while he himself was drowning in the ocean of our loss. My amazing son Benjamin, for bringing color back into my world and saving my life just by being here. And Nathaniel, the tiny baby boy that is growing inside of me as I sit here writing, for reminding me that there is still hope and joy in my heart.

To the amazing community of bereaved parents that I have met while traveling this new path, especially the DS Moms, you have reminded me that I am not crazy and I am not alone. I wish none of us ever had a reason to meet, but I am thankful that we have found each other.

And to Beth, Joanna, Catherine & Amy: you have been my strength and my sanity. I will be forever grateful.

Contents

Foreword

Generations ago it was a different culture for families whose babies died. They were silenced immediately upon giving birth to their dead children. They often did not see the child. They were told it was abnormal to name the child. There were usually no rituals performed, though there may have been a gravesite and stone to mark the otherwise silenced experience. Families were certainly not encouraged to visit the grave regularly. There were no support groups for these families. I cannot tell you how many women of my grandmother's age have told me how they lived isolated and alone with the full truth of their motherhood. The motherhood that included having given birth to death. The truth of a family tree that was missing the name of the child who died.

Today things are different. We have the example of protesters and rights movements and model advocates to thank for the fact that we can choose a different reality today. On the shoulders of grief advocates like Dr. Elisabeth Kubler-Ross, Dr. John DeFrain, Dr. Joanne Cacciatore, filmmaker Vanessa Gorman, families like ours have a choice to speak up, speak out, advocate for our own best care, and for the compassionate care of other families who must endure the death of a child.

Stephanie Cole is another leader, another outstanding model for how we can become grief advocates. In the pages that follow, she does not hesitate to share every moment of the journey with us. She stands at the dark abyss between what she wanted and what she now faced after the death of her baby. She fully expressed the chaos and destruction of grief and found that the shards created a mosaic of a fully felt life. She embraced the full field of her motherhood as protector, provider, advocate for *all* her children, both living and dead. She braved standing by her partner as they each found their way through the abyss and discovered new ways of reaching each other even as they expressed grief differently, individually.

As we work together to change the culture of grief and parenthood for the generations to come, books like "Still." model for us how we can creatively find a liberated way to experience the births and deaths of our children. Not only do we change the culture for the next generation, but we provide safe space for our grandmothers' generation to speak up now, too. "Still." shows us how look at grief and our different kind of parenting even when we feel overwhelmed by the chaos. Stephanie models for us how to journal, paint, sculpt, shatter, glue together, take a poetic view. All of these are tools we can use to look askew and try to get a handle on our experience when looking straight on is just too much. Stephanie does not prescribe one single way. She does not claim to have the fix or the exact path we must all adhere to. But rather she shares all the tools she used. She gives you the choice to try what feels right to you. She models one way and leaves all the other branches off the path open for you to try as you need and want.

This book and Stephanie's work are part of the lineage of advocacy. From hospice to Compassionate Friends, from Tear Soup to the Centering Corporation, from MISS Foundation to SHARE, from Dear Cheyenne to Losing Layla. Stephanie's words show us clearly that though our birth experiences are different than most, our parenthood and the love we have for our children, "Still." to this day, remain.

Kara L.C. Jones, 2010
Grief & Creativity Coach at MotherHenna.com

Introduction

This book is not something that I wrote as much as it is something that grew from me, from my grief. When my daughter died unexpectedly it shook me to my very core. I kept a journal throughout my pregnancy, and it seemed natural to continue afterward. I had a hard time falling asleep at night, and I found that if I purged my emotions onto the pages of my journal right before bed I was able to fall asleep easier. I also found painting and sculpting to be great outlets for all the heartache and frustration that had taken hold of me. I put this book together as a way to reach out to other parents who are facing this unimaginable loss. After Madeline died, I felt like I was the only person in the world who had suffered through this. It is such a lonely loss. It is my hope that a mother (or father or sibling or grandparent) may find something in this book that speaks to her own broken heart. That something I wrote or painted makes her nod her head and sigh, and hopefully feel a little less alone.

Thursday

Concerned
Nervous
Anxious
Uncertain
Concerned
Why are they worried?
What's going on?
Kind of excited
I love ultrasounds
Is something wrong?
Their faces are frozen
Worried, just a little
BAM
"I'm so sorry . . ."
She's dead
It washes over me
Drags me under
She's dead
She's dead
Dizzy
Disbelief
No
NO
Do it again
They turn the monitor
I look
But I can't see
I'm gone
So is she

Dizzy
Dizzy
Nothing makes sense
"Wait here"
"Richy's coming"
"Here is a gown"
No
NO
I stay in my clothes
He's here
He's crying
Now I can cry
Maybe I'll kill myself
I wish I knew how
Confused
Scared
Complete disbelief
What are they asking of me?
I have to labor?
She needs to come out?
No
NO
This is all wrong
I want to go home
I want to die
Please make it stop
Why won't it just stop?
Silence
Resolve
Utter disbelief
I detach from my body
They do things to that girl
I guess that she's me
IV, Pitocin, catheter
I don't care
Water breaks
Muscles contract

I don't feel them
Are they even mine?
Baby is coming
One last push
No
I won't
You'll take her from me
Keep her inside
She's safe with her mommy
No choice
No control
My body betrays me
She's out
She is dead
They say "it was a girl"
Has she stopped being one?
She is a girl
I know
She's my daughter
I hold her
I love her
They take her away
I fall
Down
Down
Down
Days pass
Shock lifts
Disbelief stays
Pain comes
Piles of it
More every day
It crushes me
Darkness
Darker than darkness
Engulfs me
I stare for hours

The lights stay off
There's nothing to see
I ache
I long
I die every morning
I cry myself to sleep
I wake up
I die again
I hurt and hurt and hurt
It doesn't stop
Time does not heal
This will not heal
I will just learn to breathe through the pain
But I don't want to breathe
I don't want to heal
I just want to wake up on Thursday
And start over again

The End of
the Pregnancy

After forty weeks of excited anticipation my due date was finally here. But Madeline didn't seem to realize that this was the day the doctors had predicted her arrival, and was quite content to stay snug in my belly for a little longer. On Tuesday I went to see my doctor. He examined us, Madeline and me, and said it was up to me. We could induce if we wanted, we could wait if we wanted. We decided to stick it out for a few more days. I trusted my body, it would let me know when the time was right. Madeline would come when she was ready. On Wednesday I lost my mucous plug. Any time now labor could begin! But I was still pregnant when I went to bed that night. "This is all completely normal," my doctor told me. They were not at all concerned, and neither was I.

My pregnancy was uneventful and complication-free, and I loved every second of it. Sure there was morning sickness that lasted all day, fire-like heartburn, and constant runs to the bathroom—but the discomfort all seemed to melt away whenever I felt my little girl move inside of me. And she was an active little monster! Madeline had regular dance parties every night. She would begin to kick around 11:00pm and would go nonstop until she tired herself out. It was my favorite part of the day. Eating peach ice cream was another surefire way to get her going. A few bites and she was kicking up a storm. Madeline also had very predictable hiccups every morning right around 8:00am. Her hiccups were so predictable that I eventually stopped setting an alarm clock, relying completely on Madeline to hiccup me awake every morning. On Wednesday night, after her dance party, my husband read Maddie her bedtime story, just like he had every night since we first found out I was pregnant. After the story we got ready for bed. He gave me a hug and Madeline kicked me so hard that he felt it through my belly into his, and we joked that she was jealous of me hugging her Daddy. That was the last time either of us felt her kick. I woke up to unusual movement a few hours later. It felt like Madeline was twitching. I woke Richy up and we considered going to the hospital. The twitching stopped, and I wasn't cramping or anything, so we went back to bed.

On Thursday I didn't wake up until after 10:00am. No hiccups. That should have been my first sign that something was wrong. I ate ice cream for breakfast, hoping that the sugar rush would get her moving. I had heard that babies tend to slow down a bit right before birth, so I thought maybe labor was about to begin. I took a shower and rubbed my belly and sang to Madeline. Nothing. I was getting pretty nervous as I got out of the shower, and was on the phone with the nurse from maternal fetal medicine before I had even gotten dressed. She said I should come in just to get checked out, just to ease my mind. I called my husband as I was getting dressed, he said he was sure that everything was fine but that I could call him if I needed and he would leave work right away. I called my mom to let her know that I was going to the hospital. She offered to meet me there, but I told her there was no need for that, I would just call her later and let her know how things went. I grabbed my pillow and the camcorder, just in case I did end up going into labor, and headed out to the car. My hospital bags were already in the car. One bag with our stuff for labor, and one with clothes for all three of us for the hospital stay. Those bags had been waiting patiently in my backseat for weeks.

The hospital is a forty-five minute drive from my house. I spent the entire ride rubbing my belly and alternating between singing to Madeline and begging her to move. At one point I started to cry and pleaded with her to please just kick once for Mommy. "It doesn't have to be a big kick Sweet Pea" I told her, "just let Mommy know you are alright." Nothing. I stopped at a red light less than a mile from the hospital and just as the light changed to green and I began to make a left turn I swore I felt her move a little. I breathed a sigh of relief and pulled into the parking lot, parked my car and walked upstairs to Labor & Delivery.

Telling the L&D nurse that I was here because I hadn't felt movement all day made it seem more real, and a little scary, but I convinced myself that it was going to be okay. At this point my worst case scenario was that something was wrong and they would have to do an emergency c-section. My mind never even drifted to worse possibilities. After forty-one weeks of problem-free pregnancy, I thought Madeline was a sure thing. The nurse had me give a urine sample and then led me to a small room. She tried to find Madeline's heartbeat with the Doppler. She wasn't able to find it, but she said that the Doppler was acting up and asked me to wait one minute while she got the ultrasound machine. My mom walked in just as she was about to do the ultrasound. My mom is such a good mom. I am eternally grateful to her for ignoring me and coming anyway. The nurse began to do the ultrasound, but stopped after just a few seconds. She turned off the monitor and again blamed the machine. This ultrasound machine is so old and useless, was the lie she used. She told me she would take me across the hall to a newer machine, she just had to go make sure it was available. When she left the room my mom looked at me with worried eyes, she looked so much more worried than I was. She said she thought we should call Richy, that he needs to come now, and she stepped out into the hallway to call him. They took me across the hallway and I was still so oblivious to what was about to happen that when we walked into the room, I smiled. This was the same room where we first learned that Madeline was a little girl. I loved this room.

The head of maternal fetal medicine came in to do the ultrasound, along with the attending nurse. They had been the
ones to follow me throughout my pregnancy, so it was nice
to see faces I knew. The nurse stood by my side and I noticed
that she looked very worried. I asked her if everything was
okay, if she thought something was really wrong. She told me
that they just wanted to be sure, but didn't really make eye
contact. She must have already known. I think by that point,
everyone knew but me. The doctor began the ultrasound and
turned to me, "I'm sorry Mrs. Cole, the baby is gone."

It didn't make sense to me. I told him no. I told him to do
it again. He put the wand back on my belly and turned the
screen to me. He pointed to her heart. It was still. I have no
memory of seeing it though, I think I had lost my vision by
that point. I had also lost my ability to process information. I
felt like I was falling, I was dizzy, I couldn't breathe. I didn't
want to breathe. Nothing made sense. The nurse began crying and my mom rushed over to me and started stroking my
hair and talking to me. I pushed them both away and, trying
desperately to get hold of myself and remain calm, I turned to
the doctor and said, "Okay, so what can we do now? What do
we do?" He looked at me sympathetically and began talking
to me quietly and gently about inducing labor. Oh my God,
I still have to give birth?!? "No, no. We need to fix this. How
do we fix this? How do we get her back? What can I do?"
Everyone just stood there looking at me with such sadness,
offering me nothing but their own tears and broken hearts.
Still lying on the ultrasound bed with goo all over my belly,
I took my mom's cell phone and called Richy. I was so con-
sumed by shock and disbelief that when he answered I just
flatly said, "She's gone. Madeline's dead." Then I handed the
phone back to my mom. I wasn't the only one who couldn't
process the truth. My mom had to repeat it a dozen times before Richy stopped saying, "Wait, what?" He was in a car with
a co-worker about an hour away from the hospital. His co-

worker immediately began driving to the hospital, with Richy sobbing uncontrollably the entire way.

Back at the hospital, someone had led me to a small windowless room somewhere in the L&D wing. I don't remember getting off the ultrasound bed or walking to the room. I only remember being there. I do remember someone handing me a gown and telling me to change into it, but I refused. I just sat on the bed, completely still and silent, and stared at the walls. My mom stood motionless nearby. At one point I told her I was going to kill myself. She closed her eyes and whispered, "I know." When Richy finally arrived our doctor was waiting for him at the elevator. He brought him to my tiny corner of hell and left us alone for awhile. My mom stepped out and Richy and I collapsed into each other and cried and cried and cried.

Eventually it was time to move to a Labor & Delivery room and begin the induction. It was about 7:00pm at that point. My body was shaking so hard that they had difficulty putting in the IV and getting everything started. They gave me blankets, but the chill was coming from inside. No amount of blankets could warm me, nothing could stop my shaking. When I started to feel contractions they gave me an epidural. They didn't want me to have to feel pain. I couldn't have cared less about contractions at that point. I was numb. I was dead. Richy lay on a cot next to my bed. My mom curled up in a chair in the corner. Nobody spoke. Nobody cried. We all just lay there hoping to wake up from this nightmare. At one point I thought I felt a kick. Of course it was nothing, Madeline was still dead, but the nurse got the Doppler out and checked for me. I rolled back over and cried quietly into my pillow. After nineteen hours of labor it was time to push. I didn't cry out or groan or yell or any of that dramatic crap. I just did what I had to do. I pushed for two hours before they finally resorted to vacuum extraction. They told me they just needed me to give one more push and I quietly said, "No. I can't." The nurse stroked my arm and told me I was doing so well and that I was almost there, but that was the problem—it was almost over. One more push and they would take her from me. I wanted to keep her with me, in my body. I didn't want to give birth to death, I just didn't want to do this anymore. I wanted to stop and go home and come back tomorrow and have it all be different. But my body betrayed me and pushed her out. I felt my daughter being pulled from my body, and then delivery was over. It was 2:11pm, Friday January 5th, 2007. No one spoke as the nurse carried Madeline over to the warmer, where my mom helped to bathe her. The doctor gently told me, "It was a girl." Was. He said WAS. Richy was sobbing in the corner of the room. He had doubled over as they pulled her out. I looked over and saw him standing there sobbing. "I could feel my soul being pulled out of me" he whispered. That is exactly how it felt for me, only mine was physical—my daughter, my soul, was pulled from my body. He says his felt more like burning, but it was the same—she was a part of us, and when she died it killed us.

My mom walked across the room, holding her first grandchild in her arms. She handed Madeline to Richy and I watched as his face crumpled. He bent his face close to hers and whispered, "I was going to call you MadeLION." They were still stitching me up, so I couldn't hold her yet. Richy stood next to me and cradled his daughter against his chest and told her how much he loves her and how beautiful she is. Then he handed her to me. My daughter is in my arms. This is the moment I had been waiting for since before I ever even conceived, but it was never like this. I looked down at her, really saw her for the first time. She was so beautiful. What struck me most were her eyes, tightly shut but still so gorgeous—big and almond shaped like her Daddy's. The nurse later told me that they were brown like mine, I never got to see that. She had my high cheekbones and my ears, my little sister's nose. She was perfect. There is something about holding your child for the first time, especially your firstborn . . . there aren't words to describe the overwhelming rush of love that pours over you, the feeling that this is exactly what you were put on earth to do—to be the mother of this baby. All of those emotions flooded over me as I stared at her in awe. I couldn't believe that we were capable of making something, someone, so beautiful and perfect. It only took a few seconds before reality settled in. Yes she was here, she was beautiful and perfect and amazing and mine, but she was also dead. We had a few hours with her at the most, and then we would never see her again.

After an overnight labor that lasted twenty-one hours, I was completely exhausted, but I didn't dare close my eyes. It was so hard, my eyelids were so heavy and I had to fight to keep them open. I knew that this was all the time I would ever have with my daughter, and I didn't want to miss one second. I cradled her in my arms, her head resting in the crook of my left arm. I snuck my index finger into her fist, her tiny little fingers wrapped around mine. I told her how beautiful she is and how much I love her, I told her how sorry I was that I couldn't protect her. I sang "Oh Sweet Pea" and "You Are My Sunshine" to her. Sometimes I cried a little, but mostly I just stared at her. The nurse took her out of the room to take some photographs, and then brought her back to me. I held her for awhile longer, until Richy said it was time. Her skin was starting to get cold and her mouth was getting red. Her body was letting go, and it was time for us to do the same. I didn't want to, but Richy said we had to. I needed him to make that decision. If it were up to me I would probably still be holding her. We each kissed her one last time and told her how much we love her. My body shook as the nurse gently took her out of my arms and walked out of the room with her. I never saw her again.

They told me it was time to move me out of Labor & Delivery and into Recovery. Once in my room, the nurse told us that dinner was over and gave Richy a voucher for the cafeteria so that we could get some food, and then began to explain how to use the television's remote control. I stared at her blankly, who cares about food or television? Nothing had ever seemed more ridiculous. They kept me at the hospital for the weekend. Richy was anxious to go, but I didn't want to leave. I wanted nothing to do with the outside world. The idea of leaving the hospital and reentering the world was horrifying. Returning home, facing her room, her crib, her clothes, it was all too much.

For a long time the sadness owned every last drop of me. I spent the first week after Madeline's death on my couch in the dark. The lights stayed off. There was nothing to see. Richy stayed home with me that first week. We both just stared into the darkness.

We had a small graveside service for Madeline one week after her death. It was outside in January, but neither of us wore coats. We were still so numb that we honestly did not feel the cold. A family friend and pastor spoke. I have absolutely no idea what was said. I was completely fixated on the tiny wooden box that was sitting in front of me. I wanted so badly to run up to it, open it, take her out and run away with her. Richy and I went up to the casket and quietly read to our little girl one last time. I read Goodnight Moon and Richy read Madeline Loves Animals, which we had chosen as her favorite during the pregnancy. Then we ran to our car and sped away. Our families went back to my mother's house and had dinner. Richy and I spent the rest of the day hiding in bed, crying and wanting to die.

Richy went back to work the next week. He needed to work, he needed to be busy. I needed to stay on the couch in the dark, so my mom came and sat with me while he was gone. I could only eat simple finger foods at that point. Cheerios, grapes, string cheese. I peeled string cheese with the precision of someone suffering from severe OCD. It gave me something to do. When I went in for my two week follow up appointment I saw a doctor I had never met before. She asked me if I was eating well. I told her I was eating, but only finger food. She looked confused. I explained that when my mother had given me a bowl of pasta I had become overwhelmed. That I just could not handle a fork right now. She looked at me like I was crazy, so I stopped telling her the truth. I gave her the answers she wanted to hear and went home and cried.

That First Dark Year

People will tell you that time heals. Those people are liars. The pain doesn't go away, you just build up your tolerance to it. It is like lifting weights. If you try to lift five hundred pounds, it is going to crush you. But if you lift it every day of your life, it is going to get easier and easier to do, and eventually you are going to lift it without breaking a sweat. I have been carrying around five hundred pounds of sad for almost three years now, and it is still really heavy, but I do have better stamina than I did this time last year.

Some people can say they've looked death in the eye. I've cradled death in my arms, in my body. Given birth to it. It's not scary when it's that close. Not morbid or eerie or anything. Just sad. Sad and suffocating.

I kept a journal while I was pregnant with Madeline, and continued it after she died. I would like to share a few of my journal entries from that first dark year without Madeline. There were many times during that year when I was certain I was losing my mind, and I was a bit hesitant to include those moments in this book. But I have come to realize that all bereaved parents encounter moments like these, and we would all feel less crazy if everyone was more open and honest about it. I remember calling up a friend and telling her about one of my grief-driven thoughts and asking her if she thought I was insane. Her response was perfect. She said, "Stephanie. A crazy thing happened to you. It would be crazy for you not to feel like this."

January 7, 2007   2 days after

They release me from the hospital. I don't want to leave, but I know Richy is anxious to go. He brings everything to the car. Then it's time to leave. I can't believe I am leaving the hospital without Madeline. It feels so wrong. It IS so wrong. They take me out in a wheelchair. I am clutching Madeline's little green elephant, I have been since labor began. I keep my head down and my hands over my face the whole way. I don't want to see anyone and I don't want anyone to see me. I feel stupid, leaving without my baby. I feel like I failed. We go out the side door and as I get in the car I see a mom and a little kid on the sidewalk. That will never be us. We speed away. I completely lose it. My belly is loose and saggy and empty. I look into the backseat of our car, there is no carseat there. We are really driving home without her. I make it through most of the ride, but get upset again as we get closer to home. Being close to home makes it seem more real. The worst part is when Richy turns off the highway at our exit. I scream. I cry. I beg him not to get off that exit. I yell and bang on the window with my hands. Then I crumple up and cry. We pull into our driveway, but I don't get out of the car. I don't even look up. I beg Richy not to make me get out of the car. I don't want to go into that house. I can't have come home without her. How is this happening? He's crying and pleading with me to just go inside. His eyes are so desperate. I don't want to make it harder on him, so I go inside. And I cry. Hard. We both do. That night I sleep on his side of the bed. It's easier to get to, but that isn't why I sleep there. She died inside of me while I lay in bed sleeping. I'll never sleep on that side of the bed again.

January 12, 2007   1 week after

I cannot believe the things I've been asked to do in this past week. I had to endure nineteen and a half hours of labor and two hours of pushing knowing that Madeline was already gone. I had to hold her for the first and only time of my life knowing those pretty eyes of hers would never open. I had to hand my baby to a nurse knowing that she would not bring her back to me. I had to kiss her one last time and feel her soft skin getting cold. I had to stay in the hospital for two days recovering, bleeding, broken-hearted. I had to leave the hospital empty-handed. I had to face her room, her empty crib. I had to pick out an outfit for the undertaker to dress my baby girl in. I had to pick a day and a time and a place for my daughter's funeral. I had to ice my chest and deal with milk pouring out because my body doesn't realize that there is no baby to feed. And I have to leave my house in an hour to drive to the cemetery to attend my sweet baby girl's funeral. How is that possible? How is this happening? How is it that forty-one beautiful, healthy, exciting weeks ended not with a happy little family, but with a tiny wooden box?

January 21, 2007   2 weeks & 2 days after
I remember the day we put the bassinet together. Richy suggested moving the hope chest from the foot of the bed and putting her bassinet there, but I said no. I wanted it right next to the bed, within arm's reach from where I sleep. The foot of the bed was too far away, I didn't want to be that separated from her. If I couldn't handle that separation, how can I be expected to handle this?

March 3, 2007   8 weeks after
Today as I was walking around downtown there was a woman next to me waiting to cross the street with her baby girl in a stroller. At first I wanted to run, but I got a grip and stood there and waited for the WALK sign. Then two older women walked over and started cooing over the little girl and talking about how it's the perfect day to take your baby for a walk. It was sunny and about sixty degrees. The snow was melting and there was no wind. It really was such a perfect day for a walk with your little girl. Needless to say, I crossed

the street before the WALK sign flashed. I'd rather take my chances with oncoming traffic than stand there watching someone else live the life I'd dreamed of for Madeline and myself. I can't believe it has been eight weeks since I've held my little girl. Life stopped eight weeks ago. How can everyone just keep on living?

March 5, 2007   8 weeks & 3 days after
Madeline would have been two months old today. I knew it was going to hit me hard, so I braced myself. I took the day off from work and society. No plans at all. No grocery shopping, no bill paying, no requirements whatsoever for me today. And I'm going for a massage. I decided I will do this on the 5th of every month for at least this first year. It's good for me. I feel connected to Madeline, I can just focus on her. I like having that time with my memories of her, away from the world. I put some pictures of Maddie in a frame my sister gave her for Christmas and put it next to my bed. I like having pictures of her around me. I know it bothers some people, but it helps me and that is what I need to focus on- things that help me. I don't want to be completely selfish all the time, but I am in survival mode right now. It's the only way I'll make it out of this alive.

I was thinking today and I feel like if Madeline was only going to have forty-one weeks, then I'm glad that I was her mother because I really treasured her so much. She was celebrated and loved throughout her short life, and she will always be honored and loved and remembered. Also, I was thinking that even though I hate so much that she had such a short life and that she missed out on so many wonderful things, that at least she never had to experience anything bad in the world. I mean, other than dying young. But she never suffered, she was never cold, she was never alone- she never knew anything except my warmth and she was always bathed in love. She never felt anything but love from me and we were always together. Not a second was wasted with dumb arguments or time apart or anything like that. She was with her mommy every second of her life. All of her time here was good. It's not enough, but isn't it something? I really think that I've come very far in such a short period of time. I'm now in a place where I would trade anything for another second with Madeline, but I know it's unrealistic to hold out for that chance. I know now that this isn't something that is going to go away. I'm not going to wake up from this nightmare. Now I need to adjust to fit this new life, this life without Madeline.

March 6, 2007   8 weeks & 4 days after
I went to the SHARE support group today. It was really good. It helps so much to see other people who are living through this, I have been feeling so isolated. I feel like I am doing pretty good normally, getting through my day and moving along through my grief in a fairly healthy way, but being in that group tonight really brought everything up to the surface. Sometimes I almost forget how real this is. I really was pregnant. I really was going to have a baby. I did have a baby. I was in labor, I delivered her- it all really happened. And then I had to bury her. I did all these things. Sometimes I feel like it all happened to someone else. In a way I guess it did. The Stephanie who was pregnant and excited to start her new life as Mommy is gone. She died with her daughter. I'm a different person. My life has changed forever and so have I. Nothing will ever be the same again.

March 7, 2007   8 weeks & 5 days after
I did a stupid thing today. I took a pregnancy test. I don't know why. I want to say that I knew it would be negative, but I guess a part of me thought maybe it would be positive and then I would be spared the ordeal of "trying." We aren't even trying yet, though we are talking about starting to try in April. Trying scares me though, I don't want to try- I just want to BE pregnant. We tried for so long with Madeline, and there was so

much heartache involved. If you try and it doesn't work then by definition you have failed, and I already feel like such a failure in so many ways. Anyway, the test was negative, of course. As I looked at it, it all just hit me. I'm not pregnant anymore. I was pregnant. I delivered a beautiful baby girl. But she's not here anymore, and now I have no baby inside or out. And if I want a baby in my house, I'll have to start all over from scratch. It's not fair! I already did this! I want my baby and I want her now! Anyway, I spiraled out of control after taking the test. I just sat on the bathroom floor and stared blankly at the wall for almost an hour. Richy tried to talk to me, but I was completely unresponsive. He was getting pretty upset, but I just couldn't care. I didn't want to talk to him because I knew he couldn't give me what I need. Nobody can. I need Madeline back.

March 8, 2007   8 weeks & 6 days after
I bought an ovulation test today. Not to use, just to have on my shelf as a reminder that there is a chance for a future someday. Anyway, the girl at the register scanned the box and said, "If you had the kind of night I had, you would not be buying this test." I was stunned. I said nothing and she continued, "My baby just cried all night long, you have no idea what you are in for." I said, "This is my second, so I'll be fine" as I grabbed my bag and walked out. I figured that response was the quickest way to end the conversation, but it's not what I wanted to say. I wanted to say, "I'm sorry, I didn't realize my purchase was any of your business." I wanted to say, "I think your comments are a little inappropriate." I wanted to say, "Shut the hell up and scan my stuff so I can get out of this torture chamber you call Target." I wanted to tell her that she doesn't realize how lucky she is to have a crying baby to keep her up all night. That I don't know what "one of those nights" are like and that I am dying inside for want of "one of those nights." I wanted to tell her that she needs to watch what she says, because you never know who you might inadvertently hurt with a seemingly innocent comment. I wanted to say,

"You could sleep soundly through the night if you had a dead baby like mine." But what I really wanted to say more than anything was, "I know exactly what you mean, my daughter keeps me up all night too."

March 20, 2007   10 weeks & 4 days after
There have been full days that have gone by without me crying. There have been strings of days without breakdowns. There have been times where I've gone hours without talking about her. I've felt normal out with my friends. I've joked and laughed. It's not a big deal anymore. I just have a dead baby, that's all. It has become a part of who I am. How did this happen? How did I get here? How am I not dying every second anymore? How am I still breathing? My heart was ripped out of my body. My soul died. How is there still blood flowing carelessly through my veins? My heart is still beating. How? Something drastic should happen after something so traumatic. All of my hair should fall out, or I should become mute or something. People should be able to know just by looking at me that something has gone terribly wrong.

March 27, 2007   11 weeks & 4 days
I have definitely entered the Anger stage. I can feel it tightening my muscles with pent up rage. It's been really nice out, real spring weather. I hate it. I feel taunted by it. It is mocking me. I feel like winter, cold and dreary. I want the weather to match. I am honestly angry with flowers for blooming. How dare they be alive and beautiful when my little girl is gone? I hate how life just goes on when the only life that matters to me has ended. It should rain every day. It should at least be cold so that people would keep their babies inside so I don't have to see them.

April 4, 2007   12 weeks & 5 days after
I noticed that I don't carry Maddie's green elephant around with me anymore. It used to come everywhere with

me, even just to the bathroom. I never let it out of my sight. Now I leave it next to my bed. When I go away overnight I bring it, but it doesn't stay with me all the time. First I was always holding it, then I started carrying it around with me in my bag, but now it stays in my room. Does that mean I'm letting go? I'm not. But I guess I am releasing a little. At first I was so clenched, holding on so tight for fear that I would fall and die. Holding on for dear life, which is odd since my life no longer seems very dear. I guess I'm more relaxed now. I still hurt really badly, but I'm not clenched quite as tightly anymore.

April 14, 2007   14 weeks & 1 day after
This is so hard. Sometimes I hate myself so much for not inducing labor and getting Madeline out sooner. Other times I hate myself for letting them strip my membranes instead of patiently waiting for her to come on her own. I don't know what happened to her, which means I don't know what I could have done differently to save her. I just don't know what I did wrong. I wish I could go back and redo it, but even if I could I still don't know which part needs to be redone. I know nothing. This is so hard.

April 17, 2007   14 weeks & 4 days after
This was the first month that we tried. We failed. It is hard not to be bitter and depressed. Part of me doesn't want to try again next month. I just don't see the point. Even if I do ever get pregnant, that isn't a guarantee that I'll have a baby. I've learned the hard way that pregnancy doesn't always equal baby. Don't tell me that won't happen again. Don't tell me everything will be fine this time. That isn't a promise that anyone can make.

April 24, 2007   15 weeks & 4 days after
One year ago today, two little purple lines changed my life forever. Two little purple lines gave away Madeline's

secret, she had been living inside of me for weeks. Those two lines strapped me into a roller coaster that was terrifying and exciting, the most thrilling and joyous ride of my life, with an ending more devastating than anybody could have imagined. One year ago today I screamed with pure happiness when I found out I was going to be a mommy. I knew it would be a challenge. I never dreamed it would be like this.

April 26, 2007   15 weeks & 6 days after

It's raining hard outside. The first big rain of the spring. No thunder yet, but very hard rain. I wonder what Madeline would think of it. Would she sleep right through it, or would the storm scare her? I know so little about her. Today was rough, I was completely blind sided. An artist at the gallery asked me how my baby was doing. I guess nobody told him. He was clearly upset and very apologetic, stumbling all over himself. The worst part was that he was at the studio with his two little girls and very pregnant wife. I left work soon after that. The storm is getting really heavy now. Lots of thunder and lightning. I bet it wouldn't bother Madeline.

April 28, 2007   16 weeks & 1 day after

I went to see my little brother's school play tonight. I just kept thinking about how great it would be if while I was there, Richy and Madeline were playing together at home. I would call during intermission to check on them, and of course Richy would have it all under control but I would still be nervous leaving my baby. It would be so nice, they would have Daddy and Maddie time, and I would come home to find them playing on the floor together. I had this whole fantasy in my head as I drove home. When I got home I just sat in the driveway with my head on the steering wheel for a long time. Finally I forced myself to go inside and re-enter reality.

May 5, 2007   17 weeks & 1 day after
Madeline would be four months old today. Four months.
All in all today wasn't too terrible. I had my massage at 11am.
Then Richy and I went to the nursery and bought plants for
the garden. The majority of the day was spent planting Madeline's Garden. So far I've planted forget-me-nots and zinnias.
I put glass stones in the dirt around the flowers. I like how it
turned out. Working on it was a really good way to get through
the day. The craziest thing happened while we were planting.
A dove fell out of the sky and into the grass between Richy
and me. It didn't land, it just dropped. Our neighbor was over
and the three of us just stared at it in disbelief. It didn't move
much, just sat there for more than twenty minutes. It even let
us gently touch it with a twig. We were afraid it couldn't fly. It
was normal sized, but it still had a tiny bit of down on it. After
awhile Richy decided to put on gloves and try to put it in a
tree so neighborhood cats wouldn't get to it. When he went to
pick it up, the dove began to waddle a little. He built up some
speed and then flapped a little and before we knew it, he was
flying. He flew over the field and out of sight, just like nothing had ever happened. What was that all about? He could fly
all along? Maybe he just wanted to visit with us. I have never
heard of anything like that happening before. Could Madeline
have sent him to us? I mean, it happened while we were planting her garden on the day she'd be four months old. It seems
like it has to mean something. I don't know. Anyway, later in
the afternoon I went up to her room and emptied her drawers
into a box. It was sad, but I was ok. I didn't even cry, it just felt
like it was time to do it. Richy couldn't help me though, he
couldn't even be in the room with me. I guess we are just in
different places sometimes.
    Is it disloyal to Madeline that we tried again this month?
That I really hope it worked? Should I just be focusing on her?
I can go days now without crying. Even longer without dramatic breakdowns. Does that mean I miss her less? That I'm

getting over her? How important could she have been if losing her didn't kill me? Sometimes I want that initial pain back. I need that pain, that desperation, that all-encompassing hurt. It's slipping away. I'm able to think about life outside the loss. About a future without her. And I hate it. It rips me up inside. Am I getting better? Healing? I don't want to heal! I want to rip that scab open and bleed again. My daughter, my baby, she's gone and I'm alive and everything is so wrong. And it's just accepted. We're still alive. We're continuing on. It's just so wrong.

May 7, 2007   17 weeks & 3 days after
   I went to see my grief counselor today. She said she is seeing a lot of progress in me, that I have taken a lot of big steps forward. She reminded me that not clenching on to the hurt and reinvesting in life does not make me disloyal to Madeline. Still, it feels really wrong to not be so sad all the time. I'm not forgetting about Madeline, not ever, but little by little I am leaving some of the disabling pain behind. It seems as I get more stable, Richy gets less stable. He had a rough night tonight. He's lost and depressed. I try to talk to him, but he doesn't like to talk. I wish I knew how to give him what he needs.

May 8, 2007   17 weeks & 4 days after
   I can't wait until this weekend is over. I can't watch TV or listen to the radio without being in fear of commercial breaks. Mother's Day is a mean, mean holiday. Commercials have invaded the airwaves and I feel like they are personally attacking me. I'm so unsure about how to handle Mother's Day this year. I am a mother and I want to be recognized, but at the same time I want to completely ignore it. I'm going to be unhappy no matter what I do. All I want is to hug my daughter and thank her for being the best present any mommy could ever receive. I still thank her every day for that . . . I just never get the hug.

May 12, 2007   18 weeks & 1 day after
   It is official, there is nowhere safe for me to turn anymore.
In an attempt to escape reality for a few minutes, I curled up
on the couch and turned on the nature channel. There was a
show about meerkats on, and silly me thought the meerkats
would provide me with something safe and mindless for me
to watch. But no. One of the meerkats was pregnant. I considered turning it off but thought, no Stephanie, you can handle a
pregnant meerkat, suck it up. After the commercial break the
meerkat went into labor. And then she delivered her baby. Her
stillborn baby. Are you kidding me??? But you know what, I'm
glad I saw it because it really made me see that I am not crazy,
that it is the animal mother in me that feels this loss so deeply.
And you know what else, I feel more connected to that meerkat then I do to the majority of the human population. That
meerkat mom, bless her little heart, carried that baby around
with her for days and cried loudly and desperately until all the
other meerkats shunned her. The last time they showed her
she was wandering alone, crying and clutching her dead baby,
looking as utterly lost and broken as me.

May 13, 2007   18 weeks & 2 days after
   It's Mother's Day. Do I really need to say anything more?
Okay. It's Mother's Day and my baby is dead and I'm all
alone at my in-laws. That certainly doesn't help. I guess today wasn't as bad as I had feared, but it wasn't good by any
means. I hid in bed until almost noon. Richy made me a card,
but nobody else said a word about it to me. I know it was
probably because they didn't know what to say, but a little
recognition would have been nice. I went for a hike by myself
and then sat in the field for a long time. It was really windy. I
kept asking for some sort of a sign, but I didn't see one. When
I got back to the house one of the cats had just caught a baby
bunny and ran under the deck with it. Richy chased the cat
with the hose to try and save the bunny, but it was too late.

Was that my sign? That life is just plain cruel and there is nothing you can do about it? I went off by myself again after that. I started to cry. Hard. And I started to scream. I begged Madeline to come back. I told her that I need her. I begged her to help me. I screamed until my throat was raw. When I came back Richy and I went to the field and planted five fir trees for Madeline. Richy called it the Madeline Mini-Forest. It felt good to do that. Then I went and lay in bed by myself for awhile. I can't even begin to describe how I feel today. I am so angry and lonely and sad and . . . and just plain disappointed. Dead. Just horrible. I miss my little girl. But I do have to thank her. You, Madeline, gave me all that I've ever wanted when you made me a mother. It's not the way I wanted it to be, but I wouldn't trade it for the world. I love you, Madeline.

May 17, 2007   18 weeks & 6 days after
We found out two days ago that Madeline is a big sister. I can't believe I'm pregnant again. I took five tests just to be sure. They were all positive.

I miss Madeline. I want her back. I'm excited about this new baby, really I am, but it is so hard to care about anything without Madeline. She is my heart and soul, and there isn't much of me left without her. I miss her. What would her smile look like? What would her cry sound like? Her giggle? I'll never hear her say mama. I lost so much. It's so weird to be happy about this new little life and still be so devastated over Madeline. It's like I'm hot and cold at the exact same time. The hot doesn't warm the cold, the cold doesn't cool the hot. I am sincerely both. Happy and sad. Neither dilutes the other.

I think I might be a horrible person who doesn't deserve this new baby. All I can think about is Madeline. I want her back. I want both of my children, but I want her first. I want her to be two years old when this one comes. I want to go back to January and just do this whole thing over. I want Madeline to be a big sister for real. This is not how I planned for our family to be. I hate this!

June 25th, 2007   24 weeks & 3 days after
   If someone was physically as broken and damaged as I am emotionally, they would be in a body cast. People would be gentle and kind to them. They would open doors and carry things for them. They would talk in soothing voices and try hard not to upset such a poor soul. They would bend over backwards. But with me, they don't see the damage. There is no cast, no bruise, no blood. They look at me and see a normal, healthy twenty-five year old girl. Or worse, they see a pregnant girl, young and about to begin a family, ready to burst into the world of motherhood. They don't know that I've been in that world for months now, that I slipped into it silently and have been wandering aimlessly, lost and alone, ever since. I need a body cast. And a little understanding.

August 14, 2007   31 weeks & 4 days after
   Yesterday I went to the mailbox and found an invitation to a christening. I walked directly to the dumpster and threw it in. I was in tears before I made it to my front door. I'm so alone in this. Everyone else has moved on. I mean, I didn't get an invitation to the baby shower or a birth announcement, Madeline had just died and everyone knew it would be hurtful to send those things to me. But now since it has been seven months it is perfectly acceptable to rub babies in my face.

September 5, 2007   34 weeks & 5 days after
   Today was my first day of pregnancy yoga. We went around and introduced ourselves. I said that this was my second time here, and that I had a daughter who was stillborn at forty-one weeks. Nobody talked to me after that. People act like stillbirth is contagious, like I am dangerous. Like I might run over to them and touch their belly and give them "stillbirth." It isn't leprosy, people.

September 29, 2007   38 weeks & 1 day after

We bought a gravestone today. It was hell. Easily another one of the worst experiences of my life. Add it to the growing list of shit I can't believe I've had to do. We went to the first place we heard of, because we just wanted to do it and have it be done. We walked in and the woman asked us what she could help us with and I said, "We need to buy a gravestone for our daughter." I heard myself say those words and I just lost it. I went outside and cried while Richy sat down and talked with her about what we wanted and where she's buried and all that crap. Then we walked around and looked at all the stones. It was surreal. The woman showed us some of their more inexpensive stones because we said money is tight. She was very sweet. Then the owner, attempting to be helpful I'm sure, showed us stones with other people's name engraved on them and said we could flip it over and use the bottom. He also showed us a bunch of broken pieces in a pile in back of the building. I couldn't believe it. I muttered, "Why don't we just use a slab of old concrete or a wad of Play-Doh?" and walked away. I know he was trying to be helpful and work with our budget, but I was insulted. We went back to the real stones and picked out the one we thought would be best. He said, "It's kind of big for just a baby." I considered picking up the stone and throwing it as his head. Richy squeezed my hand and told the man that we had made our decision and we wanted this stone. We went inside to finish paperwork and tell them what we wanted engraved on it. We said we wanted a picture of a tree on the bottom corner and then we'd like it to say: Our Sweet Pea, Madeline Jonna Cole, Jan 5 2007. The woman looked up and said, "Oh, so you named her?" I said, "Yeah I did. I figured I named my cats, so why not just go for it and name my child, too." Richy suggested maybe I wait outside and let him finish up. I am sure she wasn't trying to be hurtful, she was an older woman and I know things were different years ago, but that really stung. I cried the whole way home. When we got back I just sat on the couch for two hours. I didn't read, I didn't watch TV. I just sat. I still can't believe this is my life. I can't believe that on this beautiful Saturday afternoon, after a nice trip to market, I bought my daughter's gravestone. How many other twenty-five year old girls did that today? I bet not many. I wish I wasn't one of them. Them. There is no them. It's just me.

November 20, 2007   too long after

So I had a few unstable moments this evening where I practiced the fine art of crazy misplaced anger. It was a little insane, yes, but basically harmless. I called this recreational ultrasound place that just opened nearby. I politely asked how they were prepared to handle situations where the baby no longer has a heartbeat. She said they would tell the woman to go to the hospital, that they don't deal with that because this is for entertainment. I told her I understood that, but that I doubt people will find it very entertaining to be told that their baby is dead, and that maybe they should go see a doctor. It seems irresponsible, and is probably a pretty good reason to leave medical procedures for the medical professionals. She got a real attitude with me and pushed me over the edge. I ended up telling her to rot in hell before hanging up. So maybe it wasn't all that effective, but it did feel good.

December 24, 2007

Today is just another Monday. And tomorrow? Tomorrow is a plain old Tuesday. But it was going to be so much more. It was going to be baby's first Christmas.

December 25, 2007

Today is just a Tuesday.
Today is just a Tuesday.
Today is just a Tuesday.
Richy and I stayed at a hotel the past two nights. We're on an avoid-Christmas-vacation. I got up and had breakfast,

then went back to bed. We're going to play Scrabble in a little bit, then go down to the pool and order in Chinese. Bah humbug.

December 31, 2007

Eleven more hours left in 2007. Thank freaking goodness. This has been the absolute worst year of my life and I can't wait for it to be over.

January 1, 2008

Well it is a new year. I foolishly thought it would feel different. Better somehow. That I would escape 2007 and all the misery that year had brought me. But there is no escape. The ball dropped and Richy said, "Happy New Year" and I crumpled up into a ball and cried.

January 2, 2008

I miss Madeline. One year ago today we were at the hospital making the wrong decision. I should have just let them induce me. Instead they stripped my stupid membranes and I went home to wait. I heard her heartbeat for the last time that day. The next time they put the Doppler to my belly her tiny heart was still.

January 3, 2008

I am scared out of my mind. One year ago tonight, while I was sleeping, my baby died. And now here I am, thirty-seven weeks pregnant and absolutely terrified to go to bed. I had a panic attack around 10pm and I begged Richy to let me go to the hospital and just get this baby out while he's still alive. I don't trust my body to keep him alive. And the irrational part of me, which can yell pretty loudly these days, is worried that January 4th might just be the day when babies die inside of me. I refuse to go to sleep tonight.

January 4, 2008

Ben is still alive. He made it through the night. I had an OB appointment and a nonstress test today. Driving to the hospital was hard. All I could think about was driving to the hospital one year ago today, rubbing my belly and crying and pleading with Madeline to move. The doctor and nurses remembered what today is and were very kind to us. The nurse cried with me as she hooked me up for the nonstress test. After she left the room I cranked up the volume as loud as it could go and turned off the lights and lay there in the dark, listening to the triumphant beating of Ben's little heart and sobbing.

January 5, 2008   1 year after

Happy first birthday, Madeline. I love you so much. I'm sending you big hugs, baby girl. Big girl. You are one now. You will always be my baby, though. My perfect baby girl.

I had a massage this morning. I let myself fall into a deep relaxation, focused on my breathing, and allowed my mind to drift back to the time I spent with Madeline. Then we had the Remembrance Gathering at the park where we planted her tree. Carolanne spoke and her words were perfect. My brother read something he wrote that was absolutely amazing, and we each poured water on her tree to symbolize how we continue to nurture her memory. Then we sang happy birthday and ate cupcakes. I got teary-eyed, but I held it together while we were there. Same with Richy. We cried on our own later. Everyone else was teary and sniffling, which honestly makes me feel good to see. Afterward Richy and I took a walk around the pond. It was cold, or so they tell me. I didn't feel it at all. Neither one of us even bothered to wear a coat.

I have come to the realization that "healing" is not an attainable goal. Not from something like this. The ache and emptiness and devastation and longing and desperation and all those other feelings that flooded me last January are all still very present, and can still become very intense. I'm able to function though. It envelopes me from time to time, but for the most part I've learned to live with it. And I've also learned to release the guilt. I'm not going to say that my decision not to induce doesn't still haunt me sometimes, but I do know that I made informed decisions based on what I thought was best for the health and well being of my daughter. I know that nothing I did caused it and nothing I didn't do caused it. For the most part I can accept that it simply wasn't in my control. And today I was able to get through the day by pushing all of the should be's out of my head and focusing on what is. Yes, she should be here. Yes, she should be the one blowing out the candles. But instead of dwelling on how different things should be, I tried to just focus on how things are and what I can do for her with what I have. I baked cupcakes last night, just like I would have if she were here. And her family ate them after singing Happy Birthday to her. It should have been followed by presents and so much more. And I thought about all of it. But I tried not to let it own me. I think that is as close to healing as I can hope to get. Not being rid of the devastation, but not being owned by it either. Of course it will swallow me whole from time to time, but it won't be months at a time anymore. And that is progress. This time last year I was certain I would not live through the night. Some how I've survived an entire year. Sometimes I feel really guilty about being able to live without her, but then I remind myself that the only reason I am still alive is because of the strength that she gave me. I am who I am because of her. All I ever wanted was to have a little girl, and I got her. And today is a good day, because today is that little girl's first birthday. I wish that she could be here to celebrate it, but I am here, and as long as I'm alive this day will be special and my daughter's short but so very precious life will be celebrated. One year ago today I was privileged to hold the most beautiful little girl in my arms. It wasn't how I'd hoped it would be, but it was still an amazing moment when my firstborn child was placed in my arms. I celebrate that moment today. Happy birthday, Madeline. Mommy loves you, Sweet Pea.

Beauty In
The Breakdown

I didn't set out to be creative. In fact, it was the exact opposite. I set out to be destructive. To smash and destroy.

I am a big believer in allowing yourself to feel your emotions, especially when they are grief driven. I think it is dangerous to bury them deep inside of you, where they will fester and stew until they have permeated every cell in your being. For me, I need to sit with my anger, my sadness, and allow it its space. I let my emotions crash over me and drag me under. I feel their weight on top of me, sometimes I am sure they will suffocate me this time, but the wave always recedes eventually.

In the beginning it was all shock and numbness. I felt nothing and so I did nothing. I sat on my couch in the dark and stared at the wall and ate cheerios.

As the shock and numbness wore off I was overwhelmed by the intensity of my emotions and I desperately needed a release. I would become so angry sometimes that I just wanted to smash everything in my house. After breaking some of our dishes, I admitted to my grief counselor that I was afraid I was destined for a life of paper plates and dixie cups. She suggested I buy some cheap clay flower pots and smash those instead. I bought some on my way home. Then I stood in my driveway and heaved the pots at the asphalt as hard as I could. They smashed splendidly. I loved the crashing sound they made as they shattered against the ground. When I was done I surveyed the driveway, there were shards of broken flower pots everywhere. They had been completely destroyed, and it felt good. I took a deep breath, savoring my destruction, and then went inside. My husband swept them up and threw them away. One day, after smashing some more pots, I picked up a few of the pieces myself. I looked at them and thought about how these broken little pieces used to be a flower pot. They used to have a purpose, they were molded into the perfect shape to hold a beautiful flower, and now they were nothing but wrecked little scraps. I started to cry as I thought of all I thought I was destined to be for Madeline, and how broken and useless I felt without her. I decided not to throw away these broken pieces, to instead give them another chance to be something. I collected them and brought them inside. With workable cement and paint I sculpted them into a mangled heart. This is me, I thought as I examined its rough edges and misshaped form. Badly broken but somehow still here.

Seeing how creation could grow from destruction was inspiring. And using my creativity to give voice to my emotions was liberating. I began painting and sculpting and writing out everything I felt. Sometimes I would begin a piece with a specific idea in mind, but most of the time I just sat down at the canvas with a brush in my hand and tears in my eyes, and I just let it happen. I can't even begin to explain how good it feels to release those toxic feelings from my body and spread them all over the canvas.

Turning to creative expression was without a doubt the very best thing I did for myself in response to Madeline's death. On the next few pages you will find several pieces from my Beauty In The Breakdown exhibit. It is my hope that I might be able to express my emotions and my loss to you through paint, clay, and poetry in a way that regular words do not allow.

Mother's Day 2007

I asked the earth why
and the wind whispered to me
Chaos reigns supreme

Disbelief Dreams

Disbelief Dreams of a different time
A different outcome
A different day.

Detachment Dances through my veins
Teams up with the Percocet
I no longer feel

Darkness Drowns me, I cannot see
It swallows me whole
I cannot breathe.

Death Descended on my body
It took her
It should have been me.

Gone

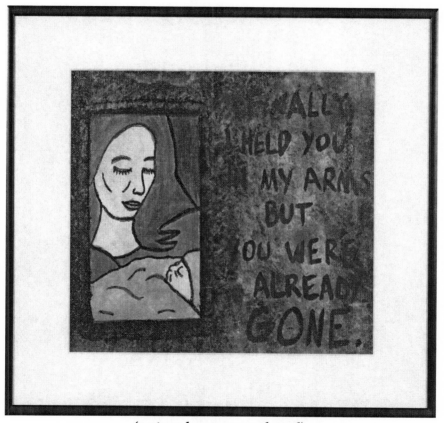

(watercolor on canvasboard)

"I painted this at 2am a few weeks after Madeline
died. It was the first time I had picked up a brush
since her death, and it felt amazing to get that
out of my body and onto the canvas."

Silence

This house is so quiet.
I hate it.
I want noise.
I want to hear my baby's cries.
It's just my own cries that keep me up at night now.

Sometimes I feel this urge,
this overwhelming need
to just scream
to break the silence.

I don't have peace and I don't want quiet.

So I scream
so loud it worries the neighbors
and hurts my throat.
But I don't care what the neighbors think.
And I kind of like the hurt.

So I scream,
from the bottom of my broken heart
and shattered soul,
for how wrong this is.
For my daughter.
For the life she never got to live.
For the lives she never got to touch.
For her eyes that never saw my face.
Pretty eyes I never got to see.

I scream and I scream and I scream.
To hurt my throat.
To end the quiet.

Empty.

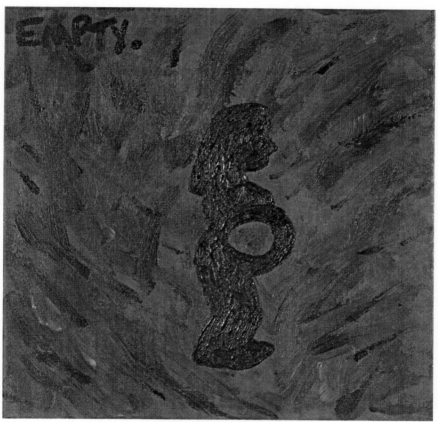

(acrylic on canvas)

"This was made very shortly after my loss, when
my body still looked pregnant, though it was
emptier than it had ever been."

(untitled I)

I know you more intensely
then I have ever known anyone.
We shared my body.
I kept you warm and nourished
and helped you grow.
There was not one second of your life
that was not spent in my presence.
I held you your entire life.
But still I feel like there was so much about you
that I never knew.
And now I'll never know.

My Mangled Heart

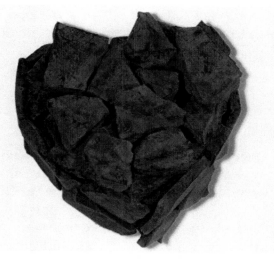

(clay, cement & acrylic)

"This piece was created from the shattered remains of the clay pots I smashed in my driveway. Like me, it is badly broken but somehow still here."

Healing Is Difficult

My belly had collapsed into its own emptiness
and blood, breast milk and tears were flowing from me
I was being drained of life
and for that I was glad
I felt I had died with my daughter
I was angry to still be alive.

But life did not leave me entirely
though I begged it to with all of my heart
And the wreckage of my body began to regain its form
The milk realized its uselessness and dried up
The blood slowed, then stopped
Only the tears continued their flow
though they seemed to drain me less and less each time.

The ache and longing are still present now
but in a less suffocating way
And sometimes her pictures make me smile a little
before I break down and cry
I guess you could call that healing
but I know I don't feel healed.

There will always be a gaping emptiness
in the Madeline-sized hole in my heart
But lately, sometimes, on sunny days
when I'm lying in the grass
and I feel the stir of new life inside of me
I realize that while I still miss her desperately
and though I still hate that this is my life
I'm not always so angry to be alive anymore.

Panic Attack

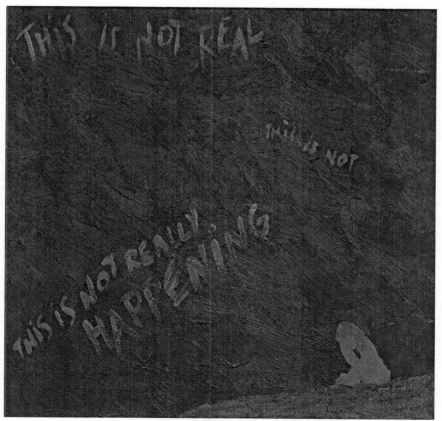

(acrylic on canvas)

"This is about the crushing force of the
panic attacks that happened when my brain
would say, 'this isn't a dream- you aren't
going to wake up' and every fiber of my
being would fight that reality."

(untitled II)

you grew in me
and I grew too
you were you
and I was me
but we were one
our lives flowing
weaving
entwined in each other
daughter
mother
connected with love
with tissue and blood
in body
and soul
and then
the end.

impossible
how can it be that one
so young
so full of life
waiting to burst into this world
slipped out so quietly
over before even one breath

you slipped away in the night
you didn't even wake me
you left me there sleeping
left me there all alone
waiting
for what would never come

Hellogoodbye

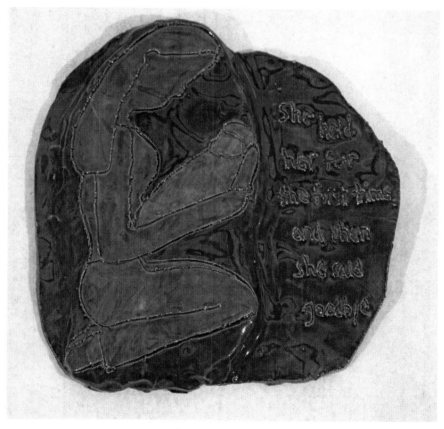

(acrylic on clay)

"She held her for the first time,
and then she said goodbye."

What Was Lost

Quiet late nights, just us two
the rest of the world asleep
I cradle you in my arms as you nurse
stare at your sweet face
and fall deeper and deeper in love
Drink in the peace of those moments
the world has melted away
For now there is only us

Later, first smiles
first babbles
first steps

You are discovering the world
and I am seeing it all new
everything is so amazing through your eyes
the grass
the snow
the rain
Take it all in
Your eyes wide with learning
And I sit and watch and smile and think
This is what life is about

This is what was lost

Expecting

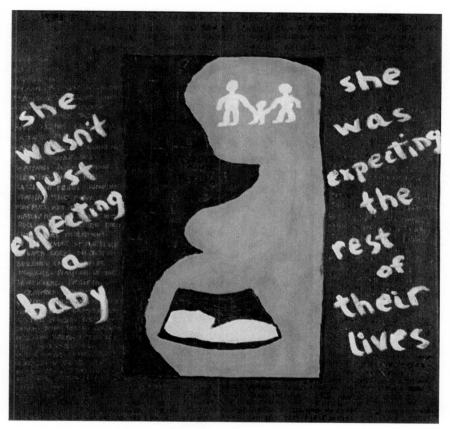

(acrylic on canvas)

"I don't think most people truly understand how
much is lost when a baby dies. You don't just lose a
baby, you also lose the 1 and 2 and 10 and 16 year old
she would have become. You lose Christmas
mornings and loose teeth and first days of school.
You just lose it all."

Skunk

my grief is a skunk.
not just because it stinks, though it does
but because everyone tiptoes around it
concerned, even fearful
that if they get too close
to me and my grief
they will get sprayed with my stink,
my sadness
and they'll never get it out of their clothes.

Response to a
Subsequent Pregnancy

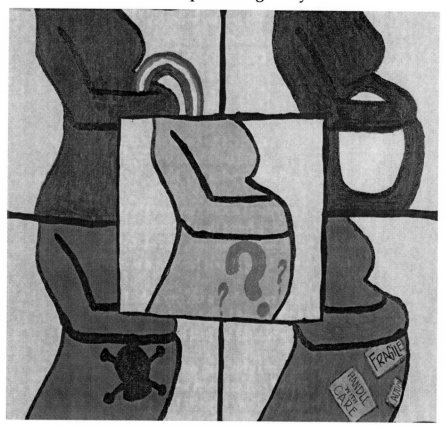

(acrylic on canvas)

"How do I feel about being pregnant again? I
honestly don't know. I feel so many emotions all
at once. I'm trying to believe in this little life,
but I know too much this time around
and I don't trust anything."

Why I Cannot Join A
Moms Group

Surrounded by women
With children in their arms
On their laps
Circling their legs

I belong and I don't

I meet the criteria to be in this club
With a little one balanced on my hip
Playing with my hair

It is a typical mom conversation
What foods have you introduced?
Is he sleeping through the night?
Anyone thinking about having a second?

That's not what's on my mind
There's a little girl laughing in the corner
She would be just her age

Now I am choking on thoughts
That I cannot turn to words
I will not allow myself to cry here

But I miss her I miss her I miss her

Talk only about the live one
You will alienate yourself
You will be the-woman-with-the-dead-baby
You will not make new friends

I repeat it until I accept it
I shut off what is real
I chat about teething
I go home and cry

Yes he's sleeping through the night
He likes pears and avocado
And we're starting to think about having another
But that would be our third.

And you don't realize how good you have it
There are things worse than sleepless nights
with cranky infants

There are sleepless nights alone

Mother's Day 2009

perfect and pretty
my sweet little flower was
more beautiful than
words can possibly describe
I'm so honored that she's mine

For Madeline

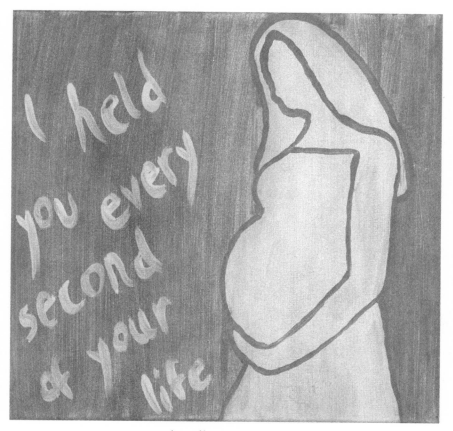

(acrylic on canvas)

"Though losing Madeline was the most painful
experience of my life, I am still so honored to be her
mother. I wish I had more time with her,
but I am so grateful for every second of those
41 weeks we had together."

The Sweet Pea Project

I created the Sweet Pea Project as a way to honor Madeline's memory and reach out to other parents who are suffering through this tragic loss. When a child dies before or shortly after birth, the parents leave the hospital with broken hearts and empty hands. The loss is amplified by the fact that there are often very few tangible items to remember the child by. One of my regrets is that I did not get to keep the blanket that Madeline had been wrapped in during the time that my husband and I held her. The Sweet Pea Project aims to keep future bereaved parents from having that regret.

The Sweet Pea Project collects blankets to donate to hospitals and birthing centers. The blankets are lovingly wrapped around these precious babies and then given to the parents to keep. In the first year, the Sweet Pea Project collected over six hundred blankets. It is our hope that the project will continue to grow so that every parent who faces this profound loss is given a soft blanket to snuggle their child in, and remember their child by. There is nothing anyone can do to take away the immense pain that comes with the death of a child, but if a simple blanket can eliminate one regret for one mom, then I'm determined to get her that blanket.

This book that you hold in your hands is another part of the Sweet Pea Project. After Madeline died I wanted desperately to read something I could relate to, and so I found myself wandering through the book store just days after my loss, way before I was really ready to face society. The selection was terrible, and the two books they did carry were on the pregnancy shelf. I left in tears. By distributing this book directly to hospitals, I hope to save parents from having to face the book store right away. I use the profits I receive from the sale of this book to donate copies to support groups and bereavement programs at hospitals.

I would like to invite you to visit the Sweet Pea Project's website, www.sweetpeaproject.org. There you will find a large library of resources, including links to websites, support groups and books that other parents have found helpful. On the Sweet Pea Babies page you will find a place to remember our children, and I would be honored to add your little one's beautiful name. There is also an online gallery that features my artwork (it looks better in color) along with the artwork and writings of bereaved parents from all over the world. I hope you will take a minute to check it out and maybe add a piece of your own one day.

How You Can Help

If you would like to help other bereaved families and support the Sweet Pea Project's vision please consider doing one of the following:

Donate Blankets

A receiving blanket would be the best. Pink or blue or neutral, chenille or cotton or flannel . . . whichever blanket you pick will be perfect for someone. We do ask that all blankets be brand new.

Sponsor Books

Purchase copies of *Still.* to donate to your local hospital or support group, or sponsor copies of the book for the Sweet Pea Project to distribute to hospitals.

For more information
please visit www.sweetpeaproject.org
and feel free to contact the author at
Stephanie@sweetpeaproject.org
with any comments or questions.

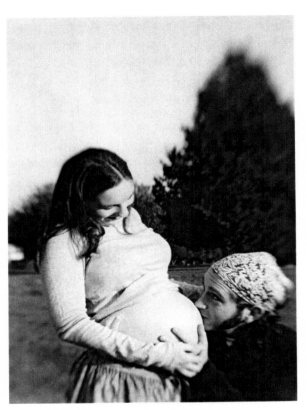

Full of happiness and life: Stephanie,
Madeline and Richy Cole

About the Author

Stephanie Paige Cole

I am an artist, an activist, and above all, a mother.

Since Madeline's death I have dedicated myself to honoring my daughter's short but precious life by working to improve the way stillbirths are handled at the hospital and in the community. Aside from writing this book and founding the Sweet Pea Project, I also give presentations at hospitals about the needs of bereaved parents, I have created workshops and art exhibits that focus on using art as a tool to navigate through grief, and I have met with senators and state representatives to urge them to pass a MISSing Angels Bill. None of this will make the death of a baby an easy thing to endure, but hopefully it will help create a more supportive and compassionate community for the families left behind.

CPSIA information can be obtained at www.ICGtesting.com
Printed in the USA
BVOW030004181012

303225BV00003B/4/P

9 781609 115869